◣ STANDARD

Acupuncture

in

Midwifery

Sharon Yelland
RN, RM, CAcC (Nanjing), MBAcC

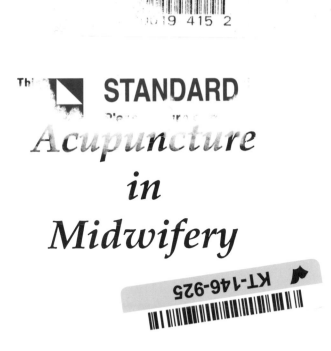

NAPIER UNIVERSITY
CB
LIBRARY

Books for Midwives Press
An imprint of Hochland &

Published by Books for Midwives Press, 174a Ashley Road, Hale, Cheshire, WA15 9SF, England.

© 1996, Sharon Yelland
First edition

ISBN 1-898507-40-6

British Library Cataloguing in Publication Data
A catalogue record for this book is available from the British Library

Printed in Great Britain by The Cromwell Press

To my late father who gave me
constant love and support throughout his life

Acknowledgements

This book would definitely not have been possible without a lot of help and support from my family and friends. I would like to thank:

- Henry Hochland and Catherine Bryant for the initial invitation to write this book and for their patience

- My mother, for doing my ironing

- Xiao Bai Li; for his art, inspiration and encouragement

- My brother Andrew, for his optimism

- Miriam Street, without whom none of this would ever have been legible

- Sarah Budd, who was my 'Vesuvius' to begin my Acupuncture training

- My dear GP colleagues at Peverell Park Surgery who keep me going

- Brian for his right arm

- and finally, all the brave women of Plymouth who never cease to come back for more needles.

Contents

Introduction

'For your walk in the foothills and glimpse at the mountain-top'

I have compiled this book with a view to help inspire and educate midwives into the basics of Acupuncture in Midwifery practice today. As it is a relatively new subject to midwifery here in the west, I felt midwives were constantly in need of information and advice from a text that was entirely related to their profession.

The book is not an in-depth study of Acupuncture in Midwifery but is more designed to be used as a guide for qualified Acupuncturists using acupuncture in midwifery or, as a 'learning-read' for midwives interested in further education and training.

The practical information contained therein has been gained from experience obtained directly from the clinical area, from treatments after trial and error and from empirical learning which have been found to be successful.

Due to the increasing interest in the use of alternative forms of healing taking place throughout the world today, childbearing women are increasingly searching for that complementary therapy which will help with their pregnancy and birth.

Acupuncture is ideal for childbirth. It gives a safe, cheap and easy to administer treatment to women during the antenatal, intrapartum and postnatal period.

Being 'drug-free' and therefore having no harmful teratogenic effects, women feel happier about receiving this type of treatment in their pregnancy. For many years midwives, general practitioners and consultant obstetricians have felt frustrated at not being able to offer women anything for the so called 'minor-ailments' of pregnancy which women suffer. For the woman, these ailments are far from minor if you have them for nine months. Acupuncture can help them a lot and make their pregnancy a much happier and more comfortable one.

At the maternity unit in Plymouth two midwives, trained in Traditional Chinese Acupuncture have treated nearly three thousand women with pregnancy related problems. The service has been available since 1989 and there is such tremendous support from both medical staff and the hospital management to continue that a third midwife has now been trained to join the team.

CHAPTER ONE

The Theory of Traditional Chinese Medicine

'It was said that 5000 years ago, in the period of Huang Di, an eminent doctor named Ma Shihuang was not only good at curing people, but also animals, especially dragons. Once a dragon circled low in the sky. On seeing Ma Shihuang, it immediately drooped its ears, opened its mouth and wagged its tail, as if in great agony. Ma Shihuang said "the dragon is ill, I'll cure it". He took out a needle from his box and applied acupuncture on its lips and inside its mouth, then gave it decoction of Radox Glycyrrhizae to drink. After treatment, the dragon rose high into the sky with all the suffering gone. Since then, quite a few dragons appeared on the mountain slope close to the house of Ma Shihuang to ask Ma to cure their diseases. One day, a dragon was seen carrying Ma Shihuang on its back, flying into the sky to some unknown place.' (Zheng, 1991).

Traditional Chinese Medicine (TCM) came out of China thousands of years ago. Yet despite what seems a mammoth period of time since the first stone needle was invented, Chinese medicine can still be used successfully to diagnose and treat twentieth century health problems today.

Thousands of years ago the Chinese were forbidden to surgically open the internal body to treat pain and disease. 'Acupuncture' is defined from the Latin *acus* - a needle and *punctura* - to puncture. *Punctura* seems to have been one of the early clues to how its success was discovered.

The origin of acupuncture can be traced back to at least the New Stone Age when the 'Bian' or 'Bian Shi', a piece of polished, sharpened flat stone or stone needle was used for treating illness by pricking certain parts of the body (Ma, 1992).

The legendary figure *Fu Xi Shi* the earliest ancestor of the Chinese people who lived in Eastern China, and *Huang Di* the infamous 'Yellow Emperor' who came from Central China were originally responsible for the invention and implementation of this 'stone needle'. It is said in Chinese history that acupuncture developed in the eastern part of the country. This evidence has been found in the Shan Hai Jing (classic of mountain and seas) which says that 'the foot of the mountains of the eastern ranges was littered with stone needles'.

From the Yin Shang period (21st - 11th century BC) a particular bone carving was discovered with the character 𤣥 which represents the ancient practice of inserting a needle into the human body (Zhan, 1986).

The period from 770 BC to 220 AD saw a remarkable development of acupuncture in which it became a popular theory and acquired systemic theories and principles. This included the replacement of stone needles with metal needles, made from bronze, iron, silver and gold.

> 'Many metal needles have since been unearthed during excavations at many places in China, including the finding of nine needles from a tomb in 1968. This belonged to Prince Lui Sheng of Zhang-Shan and his wife, of the Western Han dynasty, buried in the year 113 BC in the Bei province, North China. Four of them made of gold were still in perfect condition, but five silver ones were damaged' (Ma, 1992).

There then came reports from around China of many doctors experienced in acupuncture curing disease of which many stories are recorded, telling of dramatic and miraculous recoveries.

> 'One of the earliest stories is told of the wondering doctor Bain Que (Qia Yue-Ren) who flourished in the 4th century BC from middle - north China (Fig. 1.1) and who one day arrived in the Kingdom of Guo to be told that the Prince had just died and the funeral was being prepared. Having enquired about the cause of death and the condition of the Prince, Bian Que announced that he could bring the Prince back to life. The King ordered him to do what he could to the apparently lifeless

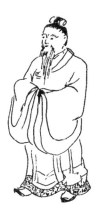

body. After taking the pulse, and examining and palpating the body, Bian Que diagnosed that the Prince was suffering from 'Shi Jue', a state of deep coma. He instructed his pupil Zi Yang to treat the Prince with acupuncture and the Prince was restored to life' (Ma, 1992).

Fig. 1.1: Bian Que

Amongst the many classics to be written following the development of acupuncture, probably the most profound works was that of the Huang Di Neijing (Yellow Emperor's Internal Classic), the earliest and most comprehensive medical work in China.

This work was said to be written by the Yellow Emperor but in fact was actually the work of many scholars and physicians living between the fifth century BC and the first century BC.

In this work, the first of its kind in the history of Chinese medicine, there is a systematic and significant description of the theory of channels and points, principles and methods of manipulation of needles, and the indications and contra-indications recorded for the use of acupuncture.

According to the Neijing, organs deep within the body, along with more superficial ones, are connected by channels or meridians through which the Qi (pronounced chee), which is vital energy or life force, and the blood circulate (see Fig 1.2). There are points on the body where the Qi of the deep internal organs lies just below the surface. These points can be punctured to cure diseases by regulating the flow of Qi and blood and restoring health.

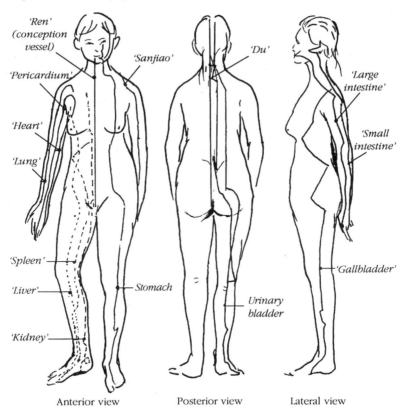

'Ren'
(conception
vessel)

'Sanjiao'

'Du'

'Large
intestine'

'Pericardium'

'Small
intestine'

'Heart'

'Lung'

'Spleen'

'Gallbladder'

'Liver'

Stomach

'Kidney'

Urinary
bladder

Anterior view   Posterior view   Lateral view

Fig 1.2: Distribution of the 14 'channels' or 'meridians'

Acupuncture is a vital part of TCM which also includes techniques such as cupping, moxibustion, Tuina (massage) and Chinese herbal medicine.

Qi

Qi is the energy or life-force of the body. It flows through the channels or meridians of the body which form a network and link all functions together. It is invisible. Its origin comes partly from our conception (pre-heaven essence); from the food we eat (GuQi), the air we breathe (Zong Qi) and from our sleep (Wei Qi). It helps to keep the blood circulating, warms the body, protects us from infection and fights disease.

In good health Qi moves smoothly through the channels, but, if for some reason it becomes blocked or too weak or too strong, then illness or pain occurs.

Diagnosis

The theory of TCM is entirely different from that of western philosophy. A practitioner of TCM would typically make a diagnosis using an holistic approach rather than looking for a pattern of clinical symptoms.

> 'The Neijing states that the body should be treated as an entity, and that attention should thus be paid to maintain the human body in harmonious balance within; and in relation to its external environment, and that the patients condition and symptoms and signs should be analysed' (Ma, 1992).

For example, we can see from below (Fig. 1.3) the type of history taken by a TCM practitioner in reaching a diagnosis for her patient:

TCM Diagnosis
• Presenting problems   • Emotional status • Family history   • Energy levels • Occupation   • Tongue diagnosis • Pulse diagnosis   • Clinical examination • Previous medical history   • Environmental factors • Diet   (housing etc.)

Fig 1.3: Presenting problems

Tongue and pulse diagnosis are very well refined in Chinese medicine. The pulse is felt at the wrist on the radial artery in three positions (Fig. 1.4) and indicate the balance of the body's energy and state of the disease, according to its strength, rhythm and quality.

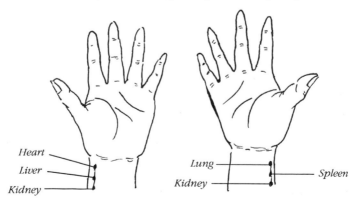

Heart
Liver
Kidney
Lung
Kidney
Spleen

Fig. 1.4: The three regions for feeling the pulse in TCM diagnosis

Dr Johannes (Bischko, 1988) in an article entitled 'Pulse diagnosis - sense or nonsense?' attempts to clarify some of the conceptions about pulse diagnosis in acupuncture. In this article he states 'it is without doubt that an experienced palpator is able to gain information by taking a patients pulse'. In summary he adds 'if the pulse gives us an answer it should be taken into consideration at least until there is a distinct change in the patients condition or renewed tests prove useful' (Bischko, 1988).

The tongue's body colour, shape, coating and moisture are also observed to gain valued and reliable clues to the patients' internal disharmony.

The concept of the interaction between opposing forces Yin and Yang is the singular most important phenomena within Chinese medicine, dating back to approximately 476-221BC (Maciocia, 1989). Balance within our life, our diet, exercise, work, emotional and sexual life is a discipline which is the key to prevention in TCM theory. Its theory is also vital in diagnosing disease.

Yin and Yang

Yin is portrayed as the dark, northern side of the hill where the sun never shines. It pertains to coldness, darkness, interior and stasis; a yin person would be described as quiet, soft, subdued and slow. Yang is the southern bright side of the hill, warmth, light, hard and changeable; a yang person being loud, excitable and hyperactive.

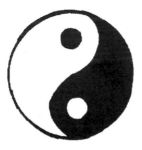 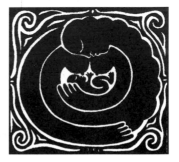

Fig. 1.5: Yin and Yang

In disease, an excess of yin can cause stagnation and an excess of yang can consume yin causing heat and an 'excess' nature.

Chinese medicine also uses what is known as the 'eight principles' to diagnose patterns of disease and imbalance of harmonies e.g. empty-full; hot-cold and excess-deficiency. A patient with a disease is then classified according to one of the eight principles or in complicated patterns, a mixture of these and treated accordingly (Figs. 1.6 and 1.7).

Symptoms	Diagnosis	Treatment
Red, hot face Rapid pulse, yellow tongue	Excess Yang	Subdue Yang Disperse heat
Pyrexia/fever Dark urine Pain 'stabbing' in nature (exacerbated by heat)		'Reduce'

Fig. 1.6: Classification of disease (TCM 'Yang')

Symptoms	Diagnosis	Treatment
Pale face/tongue - white coating Slow movements Slow pulse Thin/frequent urination Pain, 'dull' (improved with heat)	Excess Yin	Promote Yang (Warm Yin to create Yang) 'Tonify'

Fig. 1.7: Classification of disease (TCM 'Yin')

In Chinese medicine other causes of disease are related to emotional factors and are described in greater depth later in this book. Emotions are also linked to internal organs:

- Anger is associated with the *Liver*
- Sadness/Melancholy is associated with the *Lungs*
- Joy is associated with the *Heart*
- Fear is associated with the *Kidneys*
- Overthinking is associated with the *Spleen*

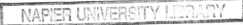

For example it has been documented in Chinese texts that too much of any emotion at any period of time can injure that organ and cause disease. External patterns of disease are also important to diagnose, and most are associated with the environment. The weather - damp, cold, wind, heat - are all influences on the state of our health. Sudden change in temperature, 'catching a cold' or too much sunshine can be harmful to our bodies and lead to disease in TCM theory.

Treatment

The client should be well received by the acupuncture practitioner at the consulting room which should be clean, quiet, warm and well ventilated.

A detailed history will follow (see diagnosis) accompanied by an explanation of what the treatment involves, its duration and the length of subsequent visits. The client should be asked to lie on a couch (this helps to ensure safety and comfort during treatment) with only the areas to be treated exposed. It is essential that the patient is as calm and relaxed as possible prior to needling insertion, as this helps to lessen the needle sensation on entry through the skin and helps to promote deeper relaxation during treatment.

The practitioner will decide on the appropriate acupuncture points to give once diagnosis has been made. Needling should be quick and relatively painless using strict asepsis, which involves hand washing, disposable needles and not handling the 'shaft' of the needle.

On immediate application of the needles or following the insertion of the needles it is important to manually stimulate the needle 'body' to attain the sensation of 'De-Qi' which is similar to a feeling of nerve stimulation described as 'heaviness', 'denseness', 'tingling' or 'numbness'. This stimulation is achieved by manually rotating and/or twisting the acupuncture needle until the client feels the 'De-Qi' sensation. This informs the practitioner that the needle has been inserted into the correct area with the desired effect. The needle may feel heavy, tight or 'sticky' to the practitioners hand once correct needling has been achieved. These are then retained for a period of 20-30 minutes.

Removal of the needles should be quick and painless - sometimes a cotton-wool ball is applied over the 'hole' once the needle has been extracted. The length of the needle depends on which area is being treated.

Advice about driving home following treatment, for example, should be given to the client (see contra-indications) as acupuncture does produce a strong soporific effect.

CHAPTER TWO

Acupuncture for Antenatal Problems

Preconception

Many acupuncturists treat women before conception in order to nourish the Qi and blood and therefore help to prepare the body for conception.

In Traditional Chinese Medicine (TCM) the two channels which control this process are the Ren and Chong. If these channels are working well the body will nourish the fetus and enable normal function throughout the pregnancy. Acupuncture can also be used in treating cases of infertility.

Antenatal ailments

There are a whole range of ailments in pregnancy successfully treated with Acupuncture in the antenatal period (Fig. 2.1).

• Nausea and hyperemesis	• Oedema
• Varicose veins	• Backache and sciatica
• Vulval varicosities	• Abdominal pain
• Haemorrhoids	*(ligamental; muscular)*
• Constipation	• Skin problems
• Headaches/migraine	• Anxiety
• Heartburn	• Breech presentation
• Carpal Tunnel Syndrome	

Fig. 2.1: Minor ailments of pregnancy during the antenatal period treated with acupuncture

Treatment should be aimed towards balancing the patterns of disharmony. However, there is one empirical point used specifically for pregnant women, Zhubin (Kid 9), which is known to block the transmission of adverse hereditary conditions. It is said to produce 'a child with a particularly luminous complexion who would sleep at night, laugh in the day time, be virtually immune to diseases or, if he/she did catch a disease, who would heal quickly, be sane in mind, morals and body' (Rempp and Bigler, 1991). 'Zhubin' should be needled once at the third month and again at the sixth month. Needling this point is also said to encourage the fetus to grow a 'full head of hair'.

The side effects of giving up tobacco or drug addiction also respond very well with Acupuncture treatment in pregnancy. The cravings diminish as do mood swings; sweating, anxiety and tremors are all improved. However, due to such high demands on the acupuncture service, such as the unit in Plymouth, smoking is often not given such high priority on the waiting list compared to something like hyperemesis or backache. Clients must be very keen to stop smoking and be prepared to come frequently for treatment too.

Some of the more common ailments in pregnancy are shown below in greater detail.

Nausea

In pregnancy this can cause great discomfort and misery for the pregnant woman and her family. According to the TCM theory the nausea may be caused by a variety of different reasons. One of the most common seen in pregnancy is called 'Stomach Qi disorder'. In TCM once menstruation ceases, the sea of blood is no longer being purged and the Qi therefore is much stronger. This then travels to and nourishes the fetus via the channel named the 'Chong Mai' - the result being more Qi in the channel together with an accumulation of Qi in the pelvic area caused by the fetus. The 'engorged' channel and the fetus push upwards, which affects the normal descent of stomach Qi, and so becomes exhausted.

Signs and symptoms typically include:

- nausea and vomiting
- weakness
- abdominal fullness
- poor appetite
- bloating after eating

- loss of taste
- tiredness
- absence of tongue coating
- cold shaking limbs

Once diagnosis is made needles will be inserted into the wrists at the point Neiguan (Per 6), Zhongwan (Ren 12) and Youmen (Kid 21) (Fig. 2.2).

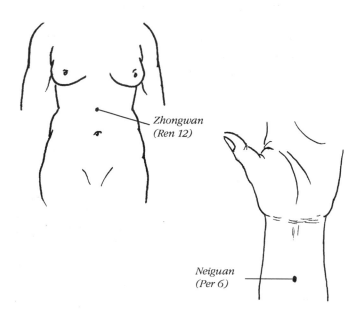

Fig. 2.2: Neiguan (Per 6) and Zhongwan (Ren 12)

The needles are rotated gently until the patient notices the sensation of warmth, distension or tingling around the needle. This gives the practitioner an indication that the needles are in the correct place. The needles are then retained for a total of approximately 20 minutes. The degree of relief from the nausea is very variable.

Some women feel much better after two or three treatments, whilst others may need a course of ten to feel that the symptoms have completely subsided. Some women are treated on the wards in the hospital (sometimes the gynaecology ward) by the midwife/ acupuncturist on a daily basis until they improve. Others are seen at the out-patients clinic at the hospital every other day or as required.

Women should be able to refer themselves directly to the clinic or be referred by their community midwife, GP or consultant obstetrician. Payment for this type of treatment is still at the time of writing, free to pregnant women.

The use of acupuncture on the Neiguan point is also very effective at relieving nausea. Research into the actions of this point with acupuncture have been carried out by Professor Dundee (Dundee et al, 1989) amongst others, with very positive results.

Women can also be guided by the midwife to purchase 'Seabands', an elastic wrist band with a central button which, when placed over the Neiguan point and periodically pressed provides considerable relief from nausea without the use of needles. This is known as acupressure.

Backache

Backache in pregnancy is possibly the most common occurring ailment besides nausea. However, it does occur at a later stage of the gestation and again responds well with acupuncture. In TCM the kidneys are essential for reproduction. The original 'source' or yuan Qi is stored here and at conception some of this Qi is passed to the fetus in order that a new life can begin and thrive. The kidney Qi sustains this growth and this depletes the maternal kidneys of vital 'essence' and is often one reason why backache troubles many women from very early on in their pregnancy until childbirth.

Furthermore, the pregnancy itself combined with the energy of the growing fetus causes an excess heat condition in which the kidney energy can become stagnated creating a 'fire'. In TCM this is referred to as 'kidney fire blazing'.

In the early part of the pregnancy the treatment is given with the woman lying prone, but as the uterus enlarges she needs to lie on her side with a pillow placed between her knees. Needles are inserted locally around the area of pain and according to her TCM diagnosis, points in the legs can also be used.

Treatment is given to tonify kidney Qi and therefore strengthen the lower back.

Occasionally physiotherapy and acupuncture are given independently as often a mechanical problem such as a displaced sacro-iliac joint is quickly corrected by the physiotherapist with good results. Some women do not have much relief from physiotherapy and then try acupuncture, and vice versa.

The number of treatments needed varies from person to person, but is usually around five or six.

Constipation

This is a very common condition seen in pregnancy responding with often immediate results after treatment with acupuncture. To demonstrate the use of acupuncture for this problem a case history has been taken from a client at the acupuncture clinic.

Case Study One

Rose   Age 30
Occupation   Secretary
Problem   Constipation

Rose came to me at sixteen weeks gestation with a history of constipation - worsened greatly during her first pregnancy. When she was not pregnant she had normal bowel movements controlled well by diet. She complained now of painful bowel movements every three to four days associated with abdominal cramps and flatulence.

She had been on various medication, one of which she relied upon totally as her only means of defaecating effectively. She was very anxious about taking any further drugs during her pregnancy but was afraid to stop them.

After a detailed history and examination of her pulse and tongue, the TCM picture was one of 'Damp Heat Retention' - probably brought about by the increase in stagnation of the flow of Qi and blood caused by the pregnancy and thus creating excess heat. This heat residing in the body for a long time turns to 'damp-heat' and causes the bowel to become 'dry' and constipation soon occurs.

After her first acupuncture treatment, Rose opened her bowels the next morning and remarked later that it had been much less painful than normal. Rose had six treatments in all and by the sixth, she was able to defaecate daily during which she experienced no pain, no flatulence and required no further medication. She was advised to come back if she required further treatment later in her pregnancy.

Contra-indication

There are some acupuncture points in midwifery that should be avoided due to their expulsive effect on the uterus. Traditionally these 'forbidden' points include Hegu (L14), Sanyinjiac (Sp 6) and Tsusanli (St 36). However, there is much varied opinion in this area depending on one's training and beliefs. Basically it is important to avoid any point which might produce a sudden downward movement of Qi, causing expulsion of the uterine contents.

Particular care should also be taken during early pregnancy or where there is bleeding or threatened miscarriage. In these cases it is best to wait until after the 27th week of gestation before using these 'forbidden' points at all.

On the other hand these points are very useful in facilitating labour and expediting delivery and can be used at a later stage of pregnancy with good effects. Zhubin (Kid 9) however is well known for its ability to prevent miscarriage and stop uterine contractions (Rempp and Bigler, 1991).

Disposable needles should be used at all times, along with proper hand washing between patients. Also, due to the small percentage of people who will faint due to a needle shock reaction or phobia of needles, the practitioner should have recent knowledge of first-aid treatment.

First aid treatment

Rampes and James in their article entitled 'Complication of Acupuncture' (1995) surveyed the literature identifying all articles referring to complications of acupuncture and have written on some of them including:

Drowsiness

This can occur during and after acupuncture, producing a potential risk where patients driving home after treatment may be in danger to themselves and others. The patient should be allowed a recovery time following treatment or advised not to drive.

Pneumothorax

There have been many reports of this serious complication world-wide. Needle insertion on the thorax can puncture the pleura leading to unilateral or bilateral pneumothorax which requires urgent medical treatment. Avoidance of needling at the nipple point is advocated amongst acupuncturists.

Cardiovascular trauma

There has been one fatality where the needle had penetrated the pericardium.

Retained needles

There have been many reports of fine linear metallic foreign bodies found incidentally on various X rays. This is usually found in clients of oriental origin who are treated by a Japanese method which involves gold needles inserted into skin permanently, the protruding part cut off.

Incidence of needles actually snapping off whilst in-situ have also been reported.

Hepatitis

Transmission of hepatitis B infection via acupuncture needles is well recognized. The use of sterile, stainless steel, disposable needles is advised to help prevent this.

The British Blood Transfusion Service screening of potential blood donors enquires about acupuncture. They state that if acupuncture has been performed by a registered medical practitioner, the donor is accepted. If acupuncture was administered by others, then the donor is asked to wait six months (Rampes and James, 1995).

Since the formation of the British Acupuncture Council (BAc.C) in 1995, which now replaces five former registering bodies in the United Kingdom, any Registered member can issue the client with a certificate which ensures that they are then not excluded from giving blood immediately. The practitioner will have MBAcC after their name.

It is also recommended that patients wishing treatment from local Acupuncture practitioners be referred to a registered member of the British Acupuncture Council (address and telephone number supplied at the back of this book) where a list of local registered members can be obtained.

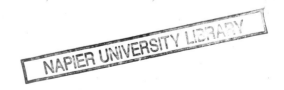

CHAPTER THREE

Breech Presentation and Moxibustion

The turning of a breech presentation using the burning herb 'Moxa' has been used in China for thousands of years. The technique is called 'Moxibustion' in Chinese and can traditionally be used to treat other conditions such as muscular sprains and pain and oedema. 'Moxa' is the Chinese name for mugwort (*Artemesia valgaris* or St. John's Wort). In Traditional Chinese Medicine (TCM) it is renowned for 'warming the Qi and blood and relieving stagnation of Qi'.

It has also been growing in our hedgerows and used in middle England for centuries and is renowned for its curative and restorative properties - place a leaf in your shoes to prevent tiredness and to 'keep the devil away!'. The herb is naturally dried into a 'wool' and rolled into a firm 'cigar' covered in tight soft paper, which produces an intense heat when burnt (Fig 3.1).

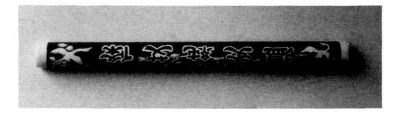

Fig. 3.1: Moxa stick

The technique for turning a breech presentation involves heating an acupuncture point on the woman's foot for fifteen minutes, twice daily for ten days (Fig. 3.2). The point used is an empirical point for malpresentation of the fetus and has been used for centuries as a standard treatment in China with a success rate of 85 to 90 per cent. It is called 'Zhiyin' or 'UB 67' and is located on the outer border of the little toenail.

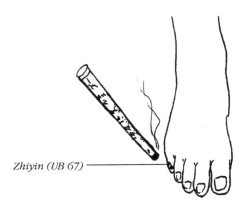

Zhiyin (UB 67)

Fig. 3.2: Moxibustion for breech presentation

In TCM the acupuncture point when heated with the Moxa stimulates and carries Qi along the urinary bladder channel to the uterus causing two main effects:

- an increase in fetal activity
- enhancement of uterine contractibility.

A western medical explanation for this suggests that the treatment increases corticoadrenal secretions, thereby enhancing uterine contractibility. This will stimulate the fetus and version is more likely to occur.

In most research papers, the ideal time for referral for this treatment is around the 34th week of gestation, therefore yielding a higher success rate. The percentage rate of spontaneous cephalic version prior to this time gradually decreases. Data available on the likelihood of spontaneous version indicates that before the 32nd week it is not advantageous to use any form of treatment to version a breech presentation (Boos et al, 1987; Golticher and Madjaric, 1985; Golticher et al, 1989).

The papers clearly distinguish between those with a high probability of spontaneous version (even after the 32nd week and before the 35th week), and those with a previous breech presentation at term, who have a low probability of spontaneous version after the 32nd week (Golticher et al, 1985; Westgren et al 1985).

Research performed in China on using moxibustion for breech presentation report a varied success rate ranging from 80.9 per cent to 90.3 per cent with an ideal time for treatment being around the 34th week gestation (Wei Wen, 1979).

In Italy in 1990 Cardini (Cardini et al, 1991) reported a 66.6 per cent success rate on a group of 33 women of gestational ages ranging from 30 - 38 weeks. This report also maintained that, as in Chinese trials, the success rate was higher in multi-gravidae, probably due to the more 'elastic' nature of abdominal muscle. As far as age is concerned, Cardini and Marcolonga, in a small trial in 1993, concluded that 'maternal age probably does not play an essential role in determining the likelihood of cephalic version during the third trimester'. In the same trial, fetal size did not seem to effect the results of moxibustion, as noted in the previous study (Cardini et al, 1991).

Sarah Budd (Budd, 1992) has completed a small pilot study, examining the effects of Moxa on maternal/fetal behaviour. The results were inconclusive but a further larger trial will be undertaken by her in the near future. There was however, a large reporting of increased fetal movement during and after the moxibustion treatment.

Opposite is an example of the instructions which are given to the women who are treated with moxibustion. After the initial demonstration with the midwife/acupuncturist the woman's partner or friend will then be shown exactly how to administer the treatment, so that they can continue at home on a daily basis.

It is important to mention here that free airflow, away from the client and attendants must be advised and ensured during moxibustion.

'Inhalation of fumes from smouldering moxa stick during moxibustion has been found to provoke tightness in the chest, dyspnoea and increased production of phlegm in persons prone to asthmatic or bronchitis attacks' (Umeh, 1989).

Moxibustion treatment

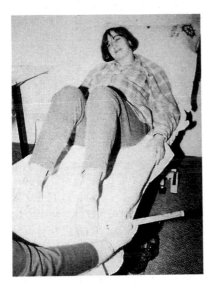

Fig. 3.3: Moxibustion

1. Sit comfortably with legs slightly raised on a foot stool and relax.
2. Light the 'Moxa' sticks until they smoke and produce a warm red glow if blown.
3. Hold the Moxa sticks about one to two inches away from the point (Fig. 3.3) and retain for 15 minutes in total.
4. The heat should be continuous and as hot as possible but not uncomfortable.
5. You may feel the baby moving a lot during treatment. This is quite normal.
6. The treatment does make you feel quite relaxed and sleepy too - enjoy it!
7. Continue twice daily for nine days. If you think your baby has turned at any stage, stop the treatment and contact your midwife or GP to check position.

In conclusion then, moxibustion is a simple, safe and effective treatment for the management of breech presentation. It is also cheap at approximately thirty pence per stick (usually two to four per course are needed).

For the future, offering moxibustion routinely in obstetrics can have great advantages. Primarily, the number of potentially hazardous breech deliveries may be reduced, and secondly, but maybe more importantly the number of routine caesarean sections in primigravida women should also reduce. For these reasons and with further research, it is hoped that midwives will be able to train and offer this technique as part of the routine treatment for breech presentation throughout maternity units everywhere.

CHAPTER FOUR

Acupuncture and Intra-partum Care

Induction of labour

In China, acupuncture for the induction of labour has been used for centuries. We know from the ancient texts, particularly the Jia Yi Jing (dated 282 AD), a Chinese Acupuncture classic, that acupuncture was used in cases of absent or prolonged labour. Furthermore, empirical points for labour such as 'Hegu' (L14) and 'Sanyinjiao' (Sp 6) together with auricular acupuncture were used routinely in state maternity hospitals in China as a way to augment labour and facilitate delivery in over 90 per cent of cases, with an apparent success rate of 70 to 85 per cent.

This method is no longer routinely used in China, as sadly tendency towards western medical methods such as an 'oxytocin' infusion is preferred. One possible reason for this is that adoption of western fashion and trends are now taking place in a more open China. Another reason could be that acupuncture in China is looked on as being slower and more time consuming compared to western methods.

Many studies have tried to explain the effects of acupuncture for induction of labour e.g. acupuncture's ability to initiate contractions prior to the woman experiencing any labour pain (Kubista et al, 1975; Ying et al, 1985; Dunn et al, 1989).

Compared to syntocinon and its possible side effects of abnormally strong contractions or rupture of the uterus (Wren, 1985), acupuncture has very few side effects or harmful responses. However, some researchers did complain that despite the contractions simulating normal contractions, it was difficult to control their intensity and frequency (Kubista et al, 1975; Yip et al, 1976). Also, it can take up to six to seven hours to stimulate contractions in some cases and may therefore be unacceptable to some women.

At the maternity unit in Plymouth, Devon, women are usually referred by self request, often desperate and afraid of the impending threat of surgical induction. This is particularly true of those women who want a 'natural childbirth' and see medical intervention as the start of the 'slippery slope' to a caesarean section. Treatment with acupuncture often helps to relax and energize the woman, even if acupuncture fails to bring about the desired effects.

Experience has shown that at least three to five sessions of one to one and a half hours at a time are necessary to obtain effective results, although sometimes one session is enough. Those women who seem to have more success are those who are multiparous and who are having some uterine activity i.e. those who are niggling, prior to acupuncture. Figures 4.1 and 4.2 shows the position of the points that are used for induction.

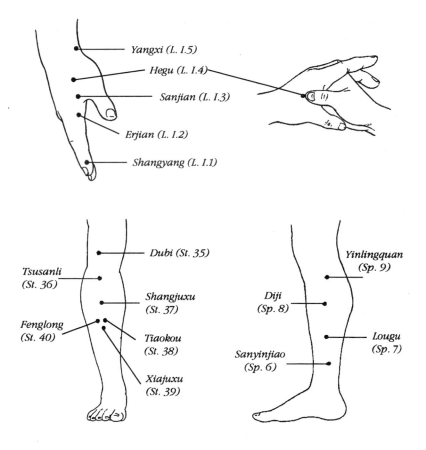

Fig. 4.1: Acupuncture points location used for induction of labour

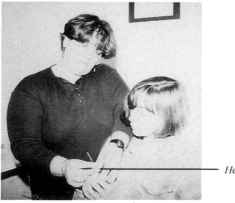

Hegu

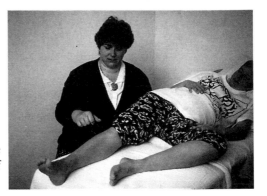

Fig. 4.2: Acupuncture points for induction of labour

An electro-acupuncture machine is then attached via wires to any two or four of these needles which maximizes the stimulatory effects. In TCM theory the points used cause uterine activity and promote a downward expulsion of the uterine contents, thus facilitating labour and delivery.

In some cases, it has been shown that spontaneous rupture of the membranes has occurred whilst having treatment. Labour will often begin that same day or 24 - 36 hours later.

'Acupressure', a firm manual pressure applied to the points, particularly LI4 is also enough to promote more regular uterine contractions, and this can often be seen clearly if the baby is being monitored with a cardiotocograph.

It must be noted therefore, that these points are forbidden to be used before the thirty-seventh week of gestation because of the risk of inducing premature labour.

Other practitioners have had experience of using acupuncture for induction of labour. Irene Skelton is a midwife/acupuncturist who pioneered the way for others with her studies on the subject (Skelton and Flowerdew, 1988).

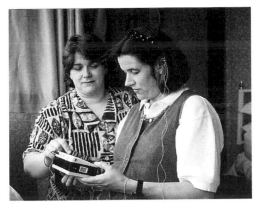

Fig. 4.3: Demonstration of electro-acupuncture equipment

Tsuei and Lai (1974) have published two research reports on the use of electro-acupuncture for the induction of labour. In the first study they took 12 women, seven with prolonged labours and five patients with uterine demise - gestation 19 - 43 weeks. Three delivered vaginally with electro-acupuncture induction only and two required an oxytocin drip.

Of the seven post mature patients, five delivered vaginally after responding well to acupuncture induction. Two patients responded with contractions and cervical dilatation but eventually underwent caesarean section for cephalo pelvic disproportion. The length of labour on average was 26 hours in primiparous women and about nine hours in multiparous women. No complications were observed to mothers or babies.

In the second study of 60 patients in total (Tsuei and Lai et al, 1977), 29 of the 34 patients term or post term were successfully induced, in that labour transpired after treatment with electro-acupuncture. Four were diagnosed with cephalo pelvic disproportion during labour and underwent caesarean section. Four out of seven women delivered under electro-acupuncture. In the seven attempts to induce in mid-trimester every case had to resort to prostaglandin induction's secondary to poor response with acupuncture. Finally out of twelve cases for treatment of pre-term labour (point 4 on the spleen meridian or Sp4) delivery was delayed in 11 women until term, giving a success rate of 91.6 per cent in this area.

Alfred Dorr (1990) used a small study of 16 women of whom 13 delivered spontaneously after the application of acupuncture using points which were known to effect the activity of the uterus. Negative side effects were nil, and besides the high percentage rate of successful deliveries there was also a significant analgesic effect especially in the active phase of the first stage of labour.

Case Study Two

Induction of labour

Susan   Age 30 years
Occupation   Television presenter
        - second baby
        - term plus seven
        - fed up and tired
        - induction with prostaglandin and syntocinon with first baby

Sue contacted me at the Acupuncture Clinic as she was going to be surgically induced at the weekend for 'post-maturity' and was desperate for a natural labour and delivery this time. She was having some strong 'tightening' and felt 'heavy down below'.

Acupuncture points Hegu L14; Sanyinjiao Sp6; Shangliao UB31 and Ciliao UB32 were used, L14 and Sp6 attached to electro-acupuncture stimulation on 30 kwz for 45 minutes.

After the treatment, Sue felt much more relaxed, but on movement felt a certain 'wetness' and on closer examination it seemed that she had had a hind water rupture of membranes.

The following morning Sue went into labour and produced a healthy 9.12lb baby girl four hours later.

Acupuncture for labour

In 1988, Irene Skelton, senior midwife at The Queen Mother's Hospital, Glasgow, reported that 'women who received acupuncture felt more in control of their labour and delivery, and were generally more satisfied with the birth experience' than the control group (Skelton and Flowerdew, 1988). Her second year study of 170 births in Glasgow investigated the comparative effectiveness of conventional analgesia versus acupuncture analgesia. The author believes that offering acupuncture analgesia to a woman in labour is a very rewarding and worthwhile experience for the midwife. It allows the woman a greater choice of attaining a 'natural childbirth' if she desires, whilst helping her to stay in 'control' by keeping her as relaxed and comfortable as possible (Yelland, 1995).

Sarah Budd introduced acupuncture for labour into the maternity unit at Derriford Hospital, Plymouth in 1988. Since then referrals have grown and today the unit has expanded to three midwife/ acupuncturists working within the hospital and on a part-time basis.

Research results on the use of acupuncture for relief of pain in labour are very variable. The main reason being the variance of methods used in assessment of acupuncture in labour, and also the subjective nature of pain itself.

In China, according to oriental tradition, labour and delivery should not require analgesia therefore acupuncture points for normal delivery were very rarely prescribed. Difficult or delayed labour however, was a common cause of death in ancient times, and acupuncture was used frequently to expediate delivery.

In Zheng Jinsheng's (1990) article 'Legends about Acupuncture treatment - of difficult labour' she records the earliest case reported from the Jin Dynasty (approximately 280 AD),

'It is said that Yu Fahai, an acupuncturist, came across a woman in labour when he was put up for the night at an inn on his journey home. The woman happened to be the landlady who had been in labour for several days, but the baby was still not born. "I can hasten the course of labour", he said to her husband, and asked him to have a fat sheep slaughtered and to make a delicious dish of it. He then forced the woman to eat more than ten pieces of the mutton. Having finished eating, the woman was given acupuncture treatment. Soon the baby was born with a layer of sheep fat covering the body'.

In the West the development of points for pain relief in labour have been prolific. In Europe the first acupuncture deliveries were performed in 1972 by Dr Christman Ehrstroem in Sweden followed in 1974 by Damas in France. In 1985 Pei and Huany of the Nanjing Municipal Maternity hospital reported on a retrospective review of

200 cases (100 receiving electro-acupuncture and 100 controls). The cases were described as having been chosen at random. However the account of the research methods used is not complete by western standards. This was due to a lack of clarity about what procedures were used to compare data from the control group with those of the experimental group. Analgesic action was graded retrospectively according to three categories based upon patient behaviour and comments. (An attempt was made to correlate degree of pain relief with type of personality but no correlation was found).

Ninety six per cent of patients received grade III or no relief from pain as compared with controls, who received no pain relief. The authors of this study concluded that point 32 on the bladder meridian (UB 32) is effective in providing analgesia in labour.

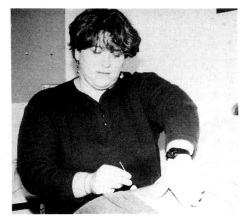

Fig. 4.4: Needling UB32 for analgesia

Later Martoudis and Christofides (1990) conducted a trial in Cyprus using a combination of auricular and hand points. The 168 participants were all in their first or second labours. A monitor was used to record uterine contractions, with the curves of the contractions marked at the point when pain began and ended. From 168 deliveries in which electro-acupuncture was used, 114 ended in normal vaginal deliveries (67.8 per cent); 42 delivered with vacuum extraction (25 per cent) and 12 required caesarean section with a general anaesthetic (7.15 per cent). The average apgar score was 9.60 at one minute which indicates a safe fetal outcome. Acupuncture stimulation varied between 20 - 30 minutes. Duration of analgesia effect was a meantime of six hours and in all participants who delivered during this time no alternative analgesia was necessary. In 24 cases electro-acupuncture had no real effect.

To obtain objective results three questionnaires were used - one to the women, the second to the midwife in charge of the labour room and the third to the delivery doctor. All were asked to scale the result of treatment between very good, medium, slight and no effect. Their study claimed a success rate from slight to very good in 87.75 per cent of cases.

Cardiotocograph recordings which were taken before and after insertion of electro-acupuncture treatment showed remarkable results.

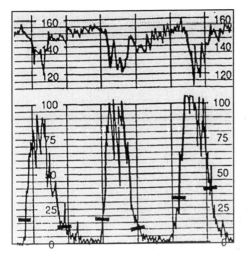

In Figure 4.5a opposite, taken before insertion of needles, we can see that pain began at the very beginning of the uterine contraction and disappeared at the end.

Fig. 4.5a: Taken before insertion

In Figure 4.5b taken when the effects of the electro-acupuncture were maximized we see that pain started at a much later stage of the contraction - i.e. near the top of the 'peak' and ended at a much earlier stage.

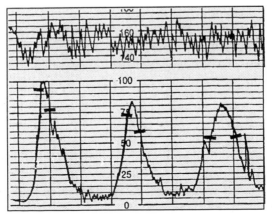

Fig 4.5b: Taken at peak of labour with electro-acupuncture

Another point that the researchers observed was that deep, fast breathing was clearly present in Figure 4.5a and absent in Figure 4.5b (i.e. once acupuncture had taken is full effect). They went on to say 'we believe that this observation is an indisputable and objective sign of the effect of electro-acupuncture in relieving the pains of labour'.

It can be seen from the ancient texts that many points which were used for the acceleration of a slow or difficult labour have been tried and adapted for use in labour for the present day experiences.

Acupuncture for labour has one problem, that of mobility for the women, especially the back points with needles that need to be retained for the duration of the labour.

In 1991 Christian Rempp recommended that the needles be inserted horizontally then taped flat to the skin. Others use points which are only given for a short duration then have to be removed. However, since the development of 'Auricular acupuncture' over the past 40 years this problem no longer exists. The ear auricle contains a complete set of acupuncture points which when stimulated can provide rapid relief from acute pain.

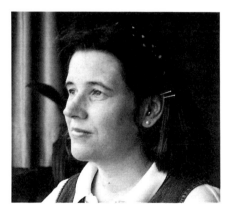
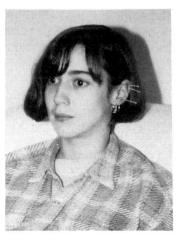

Fig 4.6: Auricular acupuncture

Nogier and Bourdiol in France along with Helmet Kropej in America and various pioneers in Japan have all worked at refining this technique with excellent results.

As can be seen from Figure 4.7 each area of the body relates to a specific point on the ear auricle.

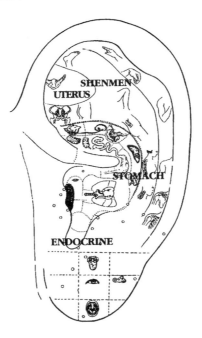

Fig. 4.7: Distribution of auricular points

The acupuncture points only become tender when there is dysfunction in the organ or limb that they represent. One can also visually compare the auricle with the normal position of the fetus in utero (Fig. 4.8).

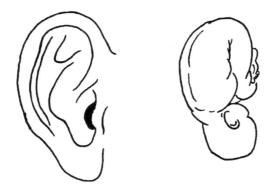

Fig. 4.8: Comparison of ear auricle with body of fetus

For labour, half inch acupuncture needles are inserted in the cartilage of the ear at the chosen points and taped down. Leads from an electro-acupuncture machine are attached to two of the needles and the woman and her partner are shown how to control the intensity button on the machine. The electro-acupuncture stimulator merely enhances the effects of the needles in situ and replaces manual stimulation. The points mainly used in labour are chosen from Uterine, Cervical, Shenmen, Endocrine, Sub-Cortex, Lumbar and Stomach (for the control of nausea in labour).

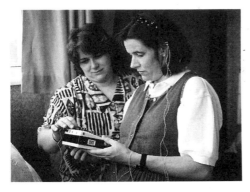

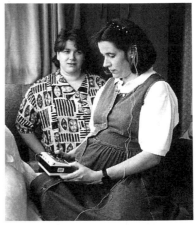

Fig 4.9: Demonstration of electro-acupuncture equipment

Once the needles are in place the woman can mobilize freely, assume natural birth positions and even have a bath (once the electricity is disconnected from the needles of course!). The effect usually takes ten to twenty minutes to build up although most women usually begin to relax instantly the needles are in-situ.

The degree of relief is very variable, some feel sleepy immediately and only 'stir' during contractions then go back to sleep. Others have a very 'active' labour. Some need to use entonox during the transitional stage of labour towards the end.

It is thought that there also seems to be a shortened duration of labour in those women with acupuncture analgesia, particularly in primigravidae.

In some women, ear 'press studs' or special Chinese 'rape seeds' can be placed on points on the ear (Fig. 4.10) so that she or her partner can stimulate the points as required.

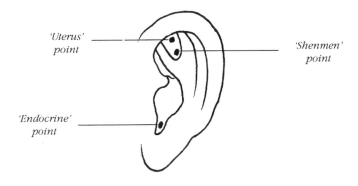

'Uterus' point

'Shenmen' point

'Endocrine' point

Fig. 4.10: Position of ear points for labour

This is quite convenient for women in very early labour or who want to stay at home as long as possible - or those who have a fear of needles.

At the maternity unit in Plymouth women can refer themselves for discussion with the acupuncturist midwife who will discuss the treatment with her and explain how it works. The woman will be given acupuncture only if there is an available midwife on duty to administer it. As mentioned previously it can be a very rewarding, worthwhile experience for the midwife/acupuncturist. However, it can also be a very demanding experience as, although the labour might often progress much faster with acupuncture analgesia, there is still a need to remain around for the woman even if another midwife is the main carer. Also because of the length of time of some labours the acupuncture may have to be abandoned due to 'midwife exhaustion'!

The ideal situation would be for all trained midwives to be able to offer this simple, safe method of analgesia to women once some formal training had been received.

For the woman who wishes to have acupuncture analgesia for her labour and delivery, it is the ideal situation for her acupuncturist to be a midwife as well.

As already mentioned the protracted length of time of some labours and the complications that may occur can give a private acupuncture practitioner many problems in the labour area. Treatment can also turn out to be very expensive for the patient, who would usually have to pay the acupuncturist at an hourly rate. Being able to offer women the 'whole package' of care as a midwife/acupuncturist can therefore add great personal satisfaction and autonomy to the midwife's practice.

Case Study Three

Labour with Acupuncture Analgesia

Cathy   Age 30
Occupation   Museum curator
               - Primigravida
               - Request for a home birth
               - Would like acupuncture analgesia for labour
                 and delivery

Cathy had asked to have acupuncture analgesia to help with the labour of her first baby. She had been attending 'Active Birth' classes, and wanted childbirth to be as natural and non-invasive as possible. Her partner Peers had also been participating in the classes and was very supportive.

Cathy went into labour in the early hours of the morning and was attended by her own community midwife, Sue. The labour was slow to begin with, with frequent bouts of uterine inactivity. However, once labour had established later that day I was called to administer acupuncture at Cathy's request. On my arrival she was coping well, practising her breathing and yoga techniques for relaxation. However, her contractions were now coming every three minutes lasting 45 seconds and she was feeling tired as she had had little sleep during the past week.

Cervical dilation was now four to five centimetres on palpation, the contractions felt strong and Cathy was concerned about her being able to cope if they became more painful and frequent.

I used 'ear' points Shenmen (for relaxing), Uterine and Endocrine with needles attached to an electro-acupuncture machine set on 'dense-disperse' at 20 - 80 KHz. Cathy and Peers were shown how to use the 'intensity' button as her contractions became stronger. This increased electrical stimulation at a time when greater effects from the acupuncture was required. Cathy was managing to breathe well and remained in an upright position with Peers massaging her back. Being at home also helped her to relax, and her progress was good. Within a couple of hours Cathy felt some rectal pressure and eventually delivered a beautiful baby girl who they called 'Ruby'.

Acupuncture anaesthesia for caesarean section

In China acupuncture anaesthesia has been used routinely for many years in the surgical area. Open lung surgery, routine abdominal operations and even brain surgery have been successfully administered using only electro-acupuncture.

When China became 'open' in 1976-79, following the cultural revolution, there was much interest from the west into the techniques of performing caesarean sections using acupuncture anaesthesia.

To date, there is no real research outside of China into this area. 'Acupuncture anaesthesia for caesarean section' states that, since 1966 5,000 operations have been performed at the Beijing hospital using the technique. Four needles are inserted to join major acupuncture points, usually along the leg and the whole anaesthesia takes about 15 minutes from start to finish.

It is claimed that the patients choose acupuncture anaesthesia as opposed to other forms of analgesia, due to it not having any side-effects on mother or baby. According to Dr Jin from the hospital, caesarean sections under acupuncture anaesthesia have accounted for 98 per cent of the total of over a thousand performed at the hospital each year – 40 per cent of which would otherwise cause anaesthesia complications.

However, at the time of writing, caesarean sections in China are not routinely performed using acupuncture anaesthesia. The exception being in several main cities such as Beijing, Shanghai or Nanjing where anaesthesia is carried out for western 'entertainment' for visiting dignitaries, or medical visitations.

It is hoped though, that in the future Britain may be amongst the first to pioneer this procedure in hospitals as a routine anaesthesia for caesarean section operations.

CHAPTER FIVE

Postnatal Acupuncture

The postnatal period can be a very uncomfortable and miserable time for some women. Below are listed some of the common conditions treated with acupuncture during this time.

Postnatal conditions treated with acupuncture

- Haemorrhoids
- Perineal pain
- Stasis of urine/inability to micturate
- Backache
- Breast engorgement/mastitis
- Anaemia
- Postnatal depression
- Back pain/shoulder pain
- Constipation
- Pain and flatulence following caesarean section
- Prolapse
- Insufficient lactation
- Tiredness/debilitation

The role of the midwife/acupuncturist postnatally is to visit the ward area where a referral for the acupuncture has been made from the woman, the midwife or the consultant. At this delicate stage of a woman's life acupuncture can be of great help in 're-balancing' the woman's energies and restoring normal health, promoting a positive start to life as a new mother.

In TCM childbirth is a very important stage of a woman's life and it is thought that a woman's vital energy can actually be improved after having a baby, from what it was before conception.

This is provided that certain rules are closely followed. For example, she must eat nourishing foods, keep warm, rest well and remain calm and happy.

In China, the woman should not come into contact with cold water but take a bath after seven days post delivery made up of ginger and red wine. Nourishing foods include chicken broth (for warming Qi and thereby strengthening the body), pigs trotters (to help with breastmilk production) and Lychee soup (to help replace blood loss).

Acupuncture can enhance the health of the woman and points can be given to tonify and strengthen the body, particularly useful after a traumatic labour or delivery.

Perineal pain

Following childbirth there is normally severe pain and/or oedema of the genitalia including the anus, particularly after a delivery such as forceps. According to TCM theory the blood to that area will have become stagnant and as blood carries Qi and vice versa stagnation of blood and Qi can cause 'heat' or 'fire' which blocks the channels 'free-flow' and thus causes pain. Acupuncture points are usually chosen on the feet or legs or both and promote the circulation of Qi around the genitalia, reducing oedema and relieving pain. The meridians chosen are usually related to the pathway they follow (see Fig. 5.1), in this case the liver channel as it travels around the external genitalia. Often one treatment alone is enough for this type of problem, but in some cases twice daily treatments are essential until good results are achieved.

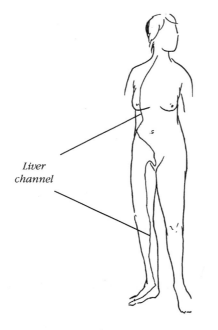

Liver channel

Fig. 5.1: 'Liver' channel to treat perineal pain

Insufficient lactation

It is known that acupuncture has a strong influence on hormone levels in the body and that success in promoting lactation may be due to an increase in oxytocin and prolactin levels. In Chinese medicine insufficient lactation occurs for two reasons:

1)   deficiency of Qi and blood
2)   liver Qi stagnation.

In the first instance treatment is aimed at promoting Qi and blood and is often combined with dieting and herbal prescriptions. As already mentioned pigs trotter is a favourite example of dieting help. Herbal remedies will include 'tonics' to help restore Qi and blood.

Liver Qi stagnation can occur due to tiredness, anxiety and worry following childbirth and this will effect the production of milk. The emotional aspect of the liver is 'anger' and this can often be seen when making a diagnosis of 'liver Qi stagnation'. The woman will complain that she has spontaneous uncontrollable outbursts of anger, accompanied with headaches and her tongue is red around the edges. Treatment is aimed at encouraging 'free-flow' Qi to the liver and therefore promoting lactation.

When using acupuncture for this problem the woman not only has a tremendous feeling of relief after treatment but usually within three to four hours the breasts are noticeably much fuller and will often leak continuously.

Acupuncture points chosen in severe cases or where acupuncture treatment is difficult to arrange, the Moxa stick may be demonstrated on Taichong (Liv 3) and the partner is then able to continue treatment at home as required.

Breast engorgement and mastitis

This is again very common in the postnatal period. Acupuncture can help relieve pain, redness and engorgement from the breasts as well as helping to treat and prevent mastitis.

PREVENTION

In China prevention is very important and advice given can be found in the 'Barefoot Doctors Manual' (1985). It suggests 'rubbing the nipples once or twice a day with a hot towel during the latter stage of pregnancy. After childbirth, pay attention to nipple cleanliness, make sure the breast is emptied at each feeding and treat the nipples immediately once cracked (may use cooked lard with the herb 'shengchi san').

The Chinese advise the use of 'cupping therapy' over the breast swelling or abscess (making sure that the cup opening is larger than the swelling). 'Cupping' involves a 'cup' made of bamboo or glass which is applied to the skin after inserting a lighted flame into the cup.

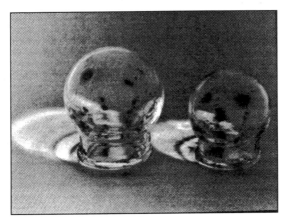

Fig.5.2: Glass inspirators for cupping therapy

This creates a vacuum on the skin and forms a tight 'drawing' sensation. It helps stagnated Qi and blood to circulate and relieve swelling and pain.

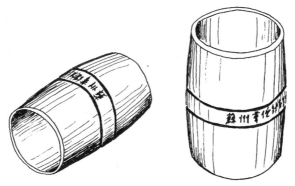

Fig.5.3: 'Cups' for cupping therapy

Acupuncture points that can be used to treat this problem can be local/on the stomach or Liver meridian. Relief is often instant following treatment and helps encourage smooth flow of milk due to its soporific effects on the body.

Haemorrhoids

Haemorrhoids can be an extremely common and unpleasant complaint in pregnancy and during the postnatal period. Being unable to sit properly also puts extra strain on the back muscles and can cause further problems such as constipation due to anxiety of defaecation.

An empirical point for haemorrhoids can be used known as Chengshan or Urinary Bladder 57 and can be found on the mid-line at the back of the calf. This point gives excellent relief and reduces oedema very quickly. Usually by the end of 20 minutes, some relief is already obtained.

For more severe swelling and pain, a point on top of the head called 'Baihui' or Du 20 is used. This helps pull up the 'yang' of the body to the head and therefore reduce swelling around the anus.

Daily treatments are given, varying between one and five in all and an appointment can be given to attend the acupuncture out-patient department for a follow-up treatment if required.

Case Study Four

Postnatal

Joan   Age 29
Occupation   Mother
                 - third baby (previous two normal deliveries)
                 - suffered from postnatal depression after
                   births of last two children - but never sought
                   or was offered help for it.

I first met Joan after she had referred herself to us complaining of backache. She was 25 weeks pregnant. She broke down in tears, and after questioning her further she did not in fact have a bad back at all, but was so frightened at being pregnant and couldn't bear the prospect of feeling like she did after the birth of her first two boys.

I arranged to meet Joan at the acupuncture clinic and after taking a detailed history from her I realized that she had had quite severe postnatal depression, which she claimed lasted nearly a year in each case.

I agreed to treat her and so we began from approximately 28 weeks up until six weeks after the birth of her baby girl.

As I was anxious about Joan's mental health I felt it also necessary to inform her GP and health visitor (with Joan's permission) that she was having acupuncture and why.

I also wanted Joan to seek help from the psychologist at our unit so that we clinicians could help 'lessen the load' and maybe offer Joan another dimension or outlet for her anxieties.

In TCM theory Joan was suffering from 'heart fire misting mind'. Her symptoms were continual mental restlessness, agitation, poor appetite, diarrhoea, insomnia with dream disrupted sleep, irritability and depression. This continued for up to a year after each birth. Her previous GP had told her she 'looked well' and that she 'should pull herself together'.

The joy of finding herself pregnant for the third time was shrouded by the dread of how she would feel up to and after her baby was born. This had already began the complicated cycle of emotions that in Chinese medicine cause the heart Qi to stagnate and 'fire' to occur. As the nature of fire is to rise, the mind thus becomes agitated and without suitable, prompt treatment, the problem does not get better or go away easily.

Joan was treated weekly with acupuncture. The treatment was aimed at calming the heart and opening up the heart and lungs allowing Qi to flow smoothly.

The points used were the wrist and top of the head - empirical points for her TCM diagnosis (see TCM diagram). These include Shenmen (H 7), Neiguan (Per 6) and Yintang (Extra).

As time went by, Joan's behaviour changed dramatically to the amazement of her husband and parents. She became more relaxed, less anxious, slept better and her appetite and bowel motions improved. She also stopped needing to see her psychologist. Joan actually never really looked forward to the birth, but when it was over so easily she was relieved and positive about the future. Treatment continued until she felt she wanted to stop and she then continued to see an acupuncturist privately during the following year - at times when she needed 'topping-up'.

The use of acupuncture for neonates

Acupuncture for babies and children has been revolutionized in this country by Julian Scott, an eminent practitioner of acupuncture. A former physicist, Mr Scott has specialized in this area mainly inspired from treating his own children when they were ill. He claims that babies, and children in particular, respond much more quickly to acupuncture than adults do, due to their greater store of Qi energy. He also teaches parents of ill or weak children to massage them according to their TCM diagnosis in order to continue the healing process at home and as an alternative to needling.

As yet there is not system to allow free treatments to our babies and children in Britain. If parents wish to have acupuncture for their child they must seek help from a Registered Acupuncturist and pay for her services.

Below are outlined a few of the conditions that can be successfully treated with acupuncture:

- Colic
- Crying
- Respiratory problems
- Convulsions
- Diarrhoea
- 'Failure to thrive'
- Constipation
- Digestive problems
- Infantile paralysis

One very common neonatal problem is infantile diarrhoea, discussed below, and how it can be treated with TCM.

Infantile diarrhoea

Infantile diarrhoea is a serious ailment of infancy most commonly seen in the summer and autumn months. It is due mostly to an inadequate milk supply, overfeeding, unclean (not sanitary) food or changes in the climate. Clinically, the most noticeable symptom is the diarrhoea itself which resembles 'curdled milk'. It may also be accompanied by vomiting, intestinal gurgling sounds and abdominal pain which causes continual crying. More serious symptoms include high fever, respiratory difficulty, cyanosis and convulsions (Barefoot Doctors Manual, 1985).

The Barefoot Doctors Manual is a health guide put together by trained lay people working in the countryside of China who are without access to immediate medical attention. In it they give firm outlines in the classification and treatment for this condition as follows.

Infantile diarrhoea in Chinese medicine has three main types:

- the moist heat type
- the appetite losing type
- the spleen deficient type

The *moist heat type* of diarrhoea is characterized by rapid onset and severity, averaging over ten stools daily, and accompanied by vomiting, scanty urination, high fever, thirst, coma and cramps.

The *appetite losing type* of diarrhoea is characterized by abdominal distension, abdominal cramps and some relief after passage of stool, foul smelling stools, nausea and vomiting, belching with decreased appetite. The tongue is yellow, thick and oily.

The *spleen deficient type* of diarrhoea is characterized by poor appetite, mental apathy, presence of undigested food in stools, cold hands and feet and facial pallor. Tongue coating is white and smooth.

PREVENTION
- promotion of nursing by mothers
- do not give infant too much food supplement at any one time
- pay attention to sanitary food habits and climatic changes to prevent exposure to cold or heat

TREATMENT
Cleanse anal area with warm water after each defecation - feed slowly and smaller amounts. Avoid cold, oily, raw foods. In severe cases reduce amount of feed by half strength feed for half to one day.

Acupuncture points:

- Tianshu (St 25)   for pain
- Tsusanli (St 36)   for pain
- Hegu (L14)   with fever
- Neiguan (Per 6)   for vomiting
- Taichong (Liv 3)   to relieve abdominal spasm

CHAPTER SIX

Training, Registration and Professional Issues

Training

In this country there are several training schools which are recognized by the British Acupuncture Council (BAcC). They are listed below.

The training in this country leading to immediate admission to the register of the BAcC is a minimum of three years (full/part-time). The British College of Acupuncture is the only one to require students to have some medical, paramedic or other practising qualification prior to entry. Prospectuses and full details of course can be obtained from:

British College of Acupuncture
8 Hunter Street
London
WC1N 1BN
Tel: 0171 833 8164

College of Traditional Acupuncture UK
Tao House
Queensway
Royal Leamington Spa
Warwickshire
CV31 3LZ
Tel: 0192 422 121

International College of Oriental Medicine UK
Green Hedges House
Green Hedges Avenue
East Grinstead
West Sussex
RH19 1DZ
Tel: 01342 313 106

London School of Acupuncture and Traditional Chinese Medicine
60 Bunhill Row
London
EC1Y 8QD
Tel: 0171 490 0513

Northern College of Acupuncture
124 Acomb Road
York
YO2 4EY
Tel: 01904 785 120 or 01904 785 828

The author's training, however, took place in Nanjing, China. There are many international training courses in China offering a three month basic and three months advanced course in Acupuncture which is organized by the World Health Organization (WHO). It is an excellent course, but extremely intensive, and not recommended if you do not work well under pressure. It takes place in China. The author advises that you firstly find out the criteria necessary for registration in England prior to deciding where to train. Extra study is often necessary in order to become accepted as a member of the BAcC. If you do train in China, at the time of writing, the newly found BAcC has only just been elected and replaces the original and registering bodies.

No criteria has yet been set as regards registration for those people who trained outside of England. For further information please contact the British Acupuncture Council.

The British Acupuncture Council (BAcC)
Park House
206 - 208 Latimer Road
London
W10 6RE
Tel: 0181 964 0222
Fax: 0181 964 0333

World Health Organization's International Training Colleges in the People's Republic of China
Beijing Association of Traditional Chinese Medicine
7a Dongdan Santiao
Beijing 100005
China
Tel: (1) 550 460

Beijing College of Traditional Chinese Medicine
11 Heping Jie Beikou
Beijing 100029
China
Tel: (1) 4225 566

Chengdu College of Traditional Chinese Medicine
15 Shierqiao Jie
Chengdu, Sichuan 610075
China
Tel: (28) 669 241

Guangzhou Institute of Traditional Chinese Medicine
10 Jichang Road
Sanyuanli Guangzhou
Guangdong, China

Nanjing College of Traditional Chinese Medicine
282 Hanzhong Lu
Nanjing 210029
Jiangsu, China
Tel: (25) 649 121 Fax: (25) 741 323

Shanghai College of Traditional Chinese Medicine
23 Lingling Road,
Shanghai, 200032,
China
Tel: (21) 438 5400 Fax: (21) 439 8290

Funding

Funding for training is possible with lots of letter writing and entry to scholarships. You need a lot of time, patience and determination and remember as Lear said 'Nothing comes of Nothing' (Shakespeare).

There have been several successful stories of midwives receiving funding for study - the author was one of them. The money was given from a local charity in Plymouth on the grounds that it would help the population of Plymouth in return.

Finding a qualified acupuncturist

A detailed list of members of the BAcC in your area can be obtained from the address given previously. The British Acupuncture Council members are bound by the Council's Codes of Ethics and Practice, and those practising in the United Kingdom are covered by a special bloc, Professional Indemnity and Public Liability Insurance Scheme. Members have the letters MBAcC after their names.

Practitioners who are not members of the BAcC may have more limited training in traditional diagnosis and in treatment (information supplied by the BAc. Council - Register of Practitioner members 12 September, 1995).

Professional issues

The *Midwife's Code of Practice* Number 40, 1993 states that:

> 'A practising midwife must not except in an emergency, undertake any treatment which she has not been trained to give, either before or after registration as a midwife, and which is outside her sphere of practice' (UKCC, 1993).

However, in the 1992 publication entitled the *Scope of Professional Practice* responsibility for professional accountability is placed firmly with the midwife rather than in obtaining academic qualifications.

The *Midwife's Code of Practice* (UKCC, 1994) offers guidance to midwives who wish to undertake further training in alternative therapies. However, there are requirements within these guidelines stipulating at what level the practitioner should be trained.

For midwives who want to use a form of complementary medicine, this means that as long as they can justify what they are doing and as long as they feel they have had adequate and relevant training, their work is within the realms of their professional midwifery practice.

Due to the huge scope of courses in the individual therapies, it would be too great a task for the UKCC to recommend a particular course of Acupuncture training. However, following the British Medical Associations report (1993) there should be some form of recognized training in all the complementary therapies. From this, greater acceptance by the medical profession is also predicted.

Insurance

Insurance is obtained upon acceptance by the Registering body, in this case the British Acupuncture Council. Further insurance is offered under the Royal College of Midwives' membership, providing that the local health authority managers are aware of your intended practice. There should, therefore, be some local policies and guidelines set down for practitioners within their area.

> 'These should ideally be devised in conjunction with midwives, managers and supervisors, educators, students, obstetricians, and paediatricians, possibly representative consumers' (Tiran, 1995).

Midwives must also be aware of the necessity to abide by other regulations within the boundaries of their profession. For example; the UKCC's publications on *Record Keeping* (UKCC, 1993), *Exercising Accountability* (UKCC, 1989), *Advertising* (UKCC, 1985) and particularly the administration of medicines entitled *Standards for the Administration of Medicines* (UKCC, 1992a). This publication specifically mentions complementary and alternative therapies and includes matters such as informed consent, practitioner accountability as the client's advocate i.e. supporting alternative therapies in relation to conventional care and vice-versa, and the right of the client to receive or decline treatment.

CHAPTER SEVEN

Conclusion

The BMA (British Medical Association) report of 1993, entitled *Complementary Medicine - New Approaches to Good Practice* set out the way ahead for complementary medicine within the health service. In it's lengthy report, a turnabout version of the 1987 recommendations, it states that doctors and nurses and midwives need to be properly trained and registered in complementary medicine prior to full acceptance by the medical profession. It also sets out guidelines for this to occur. This report must surely be seen as one of the most positive advancements for complementary medicine of this century.

Skelton and Flowerdew (1985) summarized that 'the World Health Organization sees the wealth of information favouring acupuncture as undeniable evidence that the therapy should be considered as an important component of primary health care, fully integrated with conventional medicine'.

There is no better time for midwives to be thinking about using this chance to train in alternative therapies, and use them to complement and fulfil their work. Antenatally for the 'minor ailments' of pregnancy, during intra-partum care to give pain relief and relaxation and postnatally for comfort and help with getting over childbirth.

Acupuncture is safe and easy to administer with no harmful teratogenic effects. It is easily given to women who want a more 'natural childbirth' empowering them to take control of their pain without depriving them of the 'birth experience'. It provides us, the midwife with greater autonomy in caring for our patients, without introducing harmful drugs.

Finally, we owe it to our babies to protect them as far as possible from the harmful erosions of the most traumatic journey of their lives.

'Now that many of the troubles and dangers have been overcome we must move on, not only to save more lives, but actually to bring happiness to replace the agony of fear. We must bring a fuller life to woman who are called upon to reproduce our species' (Dick-Read, 1945).

References

Barefoot Doctors Manual (1985). New York: Gramercy Publishing Company.

Bischko, J. (1988). 'Pulse diagnosis - sense or nonsense?' *Acupuncture in Medicine.* Vol. 5 (2) pp.10-11.

Boos, R., Hendrik, H. J., Schmidt, W. (1987). 'Das fetale Lagerverhalten in der zweiten Schwangerschaft shalfte bei Geburten as Beckenendlage und Schadellage. The fetal lie in the second stage of pregnancy (pregnancies) in childbirth in relation to pelvic size and presentation'. *Geburtsh U, Fraauenkeilk* Vol. 47 pp.341-345 (written in German).

British Medical Association (1993). *Complementary Medicine - New Approaches to Good Practice.* Oxford: Oxford University Press.

Budd, S. (1992). 'Traditional chinese medicine in obstetrics'. *Midwives Chronicle and Nursing Notes* Vol. 105 p.140.

Cardini, F., Basevi, V., Valentini, A., Martellato, A. (1991). 'Moxibustion and breech presentation; preliminary results'. *America Journal of Chinese Medicine* Vol. xix (2V) p.105.

Cardini, F., Marcolongo, A. (1993). 'Moxibustion for correction of breech presentation: a clinical study with retrospective control'. *American Journal of Chinese Medicine* Vol. 21 (2) pp.133-38.

Dick-Read, G. (1945). *Childbirth Without Fear.* London: Heinemann (William) Medical Books Ltd.

Dorr, A. (1990). 'The possibility of inducing labour using acupuncture'. *American Journal Acupuncture* Vol. 18 (3) pp.213-18.

Dundee, J., Sourial, F., Ghaly, R., Bell, P. (1988). 'Acupressure reduces morning sickness'. *Journal of the Royal Society of Medicine* Vol. 81 p.456.

Dunn, P., Rogers, D., Halford, K. (1989). 'Transcutaneous electric nerve stimulation at acupuncture points in the induction of uterine contractions'. *Obstetric and Gynaecology* Vol. 73 p.286.

Golticher, S., Madjaric, J. (1985). 'Die Large der menschlichen frucht im Verlaufder Schwangerschaft und die Wahrschein lich keiteinerspontanen Drehung in die Kopflage bei Erst-und Mehrgebarenden. The fetal lie during the course of pregnancy and the probability of a spontaneous change in presentation in primigravid and multigravid women'. *Geburtsch U, Frauenkeilk* Vol. 45 pp.534 -538 (written in German).

Golticher, S., Madjaric, J., Morgens, K. L. (1989). 'Mittags Bel, Ein Ammenmarchen?' *Geburtsch U, Frauenkeilk* Vol. 49 pp.363-366 (written in German).

Kubistra, E., Kucera, H., Muller-Tyl (1975). 'Initiating contractions of the gravid-uterus through electro-acupuncture'. *American Journal Of Chinese Medicine* Vol. 3 (4) p.343.

Ma, K. (1992). 'The roots and development of chinese acupuncture: from prehistory to early 20th century'. *Acupuncture in Medicine.* Vol. 10.

Maciocia, G. (1989). *The Foundations of Chinese Medicine.* Edinburgh: Churchill Livingstone.

Martoudis, S., Christofides, K. (1990). 'Electro-acupuncture for pain relief in labour'. *Acupuncture in Medicine* Vol. 8 (2) p.51.

Meiyu, S. (1985). 'Acupuncture anaesthesia for caesarean section'. *Midwives Chronicle*. April, 98 (1167), p.107.

Rampes, H., James, R. (1995). 'Complications of acupuncture'. *Acupuncture in Medicine*. Vol. 13(1), pp.26-33.

Rempp, C., Bigler, A. (1991). 'Pregnancy and acupuncture from conception to postpartum'. *American Journal of Acupuncture* Vol. 19 (4) pp.305-13.

Skelton, I., Flowerdew, M. (1985). 'Midwifery and acupuncture'. *Midwives Chronicle* May, 1168 (98) pp.125-29.

Skelton, I., Flowerdew, M. (1988). 'Acupuncture and labour - a summary of results'. *Midwives Chronicle* May; 101 (1204) pp.134 -38.

Tiran, D. (1995). *Complementary Therapies for Pregnancy and Childbirth*. London: Bailliere Tindall.

Tsuei, J., Lai, Y. F. (1974). 'Induction of labour by acupuncture electro-stimulation'. *American Journal of Chinese Medicine*. Vol. 4 (3) p.257.

Tsuei, J., Lai, Y. F., Sharma, S. (1977). 'The influence of acupuncture stimulation during pregnancy'. *Obstetric and Gynaecology*. Vol. 50 pp.479-88.

UKCC (1985). *Advertising by Registered Nurse, Midwives and Health Visitors*. London: UKCC.

UKCC (1989). *Exercising Accountability*. London: UKCC.

UKCC (1992a). *Guidelines for the Administration of Medicines*. London: UKCC.

UKCC (1992b). *Scope of Professional Practice*. London: UKCC.

UKCC (1993). *Midwives Rules*. London: UKCC.

UKCC (1993). *Standards for Records and Record Keeping*. London: UKCC.

UKCC (1994). *The Midwives Code of Practice*. London: UKCC.

Umeh, B. (1989). 'Moxibustion - respiratory complications'. *Acupuncture in Medicine*, Vol. 6 (2) p.61.

Wei Wen (1979). 'Correcting abnormal fetal positions with moxibustion'. *Midwives Chronicle and Nursing Notes* 92 (1) 103 p.432.

Westgren, M., Edvall, H., Nordstrom, L., Svalenius, E. (1985). 'Spontaneous cephalic version of breech presentation in the last trimester'. *British Journal Obstetrics and Gynaecology* Vol. 92 pp.19-22.

Wren, B. G. (1985). *Handbook of Obstetric and Gynaecology*. 2nd Edition. London: Chapman and Hall.

Yelland, S. (1995). 'Using acupuncture in midwifery care'. *Modern Midwife* Vol. 5 (1) pp.8-11.

Yip, S., Pang, J., Sung, M. (1976). 'Induction of labour by acupuncture electro-stimulation'. *American Journal of Chinese Medicine* Vol. 4 (3) p.257.

Ying, Y., Lin, J., Robins, J. (1985). 'Acupuncture for the induction of cervical dilation and its influence on HCG'. *Journal of Reproductive Medicine* Vol. 30 (7) p.530.

Zhan, J. X. (1986). 'Textual research on medicine in oracle inscriptions of the Shang (Yin) period (c.16th to 11th century BC)'. *Chinese Journal of Medical History*, Vol.16, No.1-20.

Zheng, J. (1990). 'Legends about acupuncture treatment of difficult labour'. *International Journal of Clinical Acupuncture* Vol. 1 (3) pp.309 -10.

Zheng, J. (1991). 'Acupuncturing Dragon and Ghost: Old legends about Acupuncture' *International Journal of Clinical Acupuncture* Vol. 2 (1) p.105.

Further Reading

Bensoussan, A. (1991). *The Vital Meridian*. Edinburgh: Churchill Livingstone.

Maciocia, G. (1989). *The Foundation of Chinese Medicine*. Edinburgh: Churchill Livingstone.

Shanghai, Nanjing and Beijing Colleges of TCM (1989). *Essentials of Chinese Acupuncture*. Foreign Languages Press: Reijing.

Tiran, D., Mack, S. (1995). *Complementary Therapies for Pregnancy and Childbirth*. London: Bailliere Tindall.

Index

constipation 14
contra-indication 15
contractions 25
cost 12

A

acupressure 13, 24
acupuncture
  for labour 26
  for neonates 43
  for postnatal conditions 37
acupuncture anaesthesia 35
acupuncture analgesia 34
acupuncturist 48
analgesic effect 26, 28
antenatal 10
auricular acupuncture 30
autonomy 34

B

backache 13
birth experience 50
breast engorgement 39
breech presentation 18
British Acupuncture Council 17
British Blood Transfusion
  Service 16
British Medical Association
  (BMA) 50

C

caesarean section 35
cardiotocograph recordings 29
cardiovascular trauma 16
classification of disease 7

D

'De-Qi' sensation 8
drowsiness 15
drug addiction 11

E

ear 'press studs' 33
'eight principles' 7
electro-acupuncture 35

F

first aid treatment 15
'forbidden' points 15

H

haemorrhoids 41
hepatitis 16

I

induction of labour 22
infertility 10
insufficient lactation 39
insurance 49
intra-partum care 22

L

labour
  pain 22
  pain relief in 27
  prolonged 22

M

mastitis 39
Midwife's Code of Practice 48
'Moxa' 18
moxibustion 18

N

natural childbirth 50
nausea 11
needles 2
  removal of 8
  retained 16
Neijing 5

P

perineal pain 38
pneumothorax 16
preconception 10
pregnancy
  minor ailments of 10
pulse diagnosis 6

Q

Qi 4

R

research 27

S

smoking 11
stone needle 1

T

Traditional Chinese Medicine
  (TCM) 1
  theory of 1
training 45
treatment 8

W

weather 8
World Health Organization 50

Y

Yin and Yang 6